DAILY WELLNESS JOURNAL

_____

IF YOU FOUND THE BOOK, PLEASE CONTACT:

_____

DATE _____   MO TU WE TH FR SA SU

- - - - - - - -   I SLEPT ____ HOURS LAST NIGHT   - - - - - - - -

TODAY I ATE _____

BREAKFAST

_____
_____
_____
_____

LUNCH

_____
_____
_____
_____

DINNER

_____
_____
_____
_____

TOTAL: CALORIES: [_____]

— SNACKS —

_____

WATER INTAKE ⊔ ⊔ ⊔ ⊔ ⊔ ⊔ ⊔ __ TOTAL OZ.

EXERCISE/ACTIVITY

_____
_____
_____
_____

NOTES

_____
_____

HOW I'M FEELING

☺ 😐 ☹

DATE _____   MO TU WE TH FR SA SU

┌───┐
│ - - - - - - - -   I SLEPT ____ HOURS LAST NIGHT   - - - - - - - - │
└───┘

TODAY I ATE _____

BREAKFAST
_____
_____
_____
_____

LUNCH
_____
_____
_____
_____

DINNER
_____
_____
_____
_____

TOTAL: CALORIES: [_____]

┌──────── SNACKS ────────┐
│   │
│   │
│   │
│   │
│   │
│   │
│ _____ │
└────────────────────────┘

┌───┐
│ WATER INTAKE ⊔ ⊔ ⊔ ⊔ ⊔ ⊔ ⊔ __ TOTAL OZ. │
└───┘

EXERCISE/ACTIVITY
_____
_____
_____
_____
_____

NOTES   **HOW I'M FEELING**
_____   ☺ 😐 ☹

DATE _____   MO TU WE TH FR SA SU

- - - - - - - -   I SLEPT ____ HOURS LAST NIGHT   - - - - - - - -

TODAY I ATE _____

BREAKFAST
_____
_____
_____
_____

LUNCH
_____
_____
_____
_____

DINNER
_____
_____
_____
_____

TOTAL: CALORIES: [_____]

—— SNACKS ——

_____

WATER INTAKE 🥛🥛🥛🥛🥛🥛🥛 __ TOTAL OZ.

EXERCISE/ACTIVITY
_____
_____
_____
_____

NOTES   **HOW I'M FEELING**
_____   🙂 😐 🙁
_____

DATE _____   MO TU WE TH FR SA SU

- - - - - - - -   I SLEPT ____ HOURS LAST NIGHT   - - - - - - - -

TODAY I ATE _____

BREAKFAST

_____

_____

_____

_____

LUNCH

_____

_____

_____

_____

DINNER

_____

_____

_____

_____

— SNACKS —

_____

TOTAL: CALORIES: [_____]

WATER INTAKE   ⬜⬜⬜⬜⬜⬜⬜   __ TOTAL OZ.

EXERCISE/ACTIVITY

_____

_____

_____

_____

_____

NOTES

_____

_____

HOW I'M FEELING

☺   😐   ☹

DATE _____   MO TU WE TH FR SA SU

- - - - - - - -   I SLEPT ____ HOURS LAST NIGHT   - - - - - - - -

TODAY I ATE   _____

BREAKFAST
_____
_____
_____
_____

LUNCH
_____
_____
_____
_____

DINNER
_____
_____
_____
_____

TOTAL: CALORIES: [_____]

—— SNACKS ——

WATER INTAKE 🥛🥛🥛🥛🥛🥛🥛 __ TOTAL OZ.

EXERCISE/ACTIVITY
_____
_____
_____
_____
_____

NOTES   **HOW I'M FEELING**
_____
_____   ☺ 😐 ☹

DATE _____ MO TU WE TH FR SA SU

- - - - - - - -   I SLEPT ____ HOURS LAST NIGHT   - - - - - - - -

TODAY I ATE _____

BREAKFAST
_____
_____
_____
_____

LUNCH
_____
_____
_____
_____

DINNER
_____
_____
_____
_____

TOTAL: CALORIES: [_____]

—— **SNACKS** ——

_____

WATER INTAKE 🥛🥛🥛🥛🥛🥛🥛 __ **TOTAL OZ.**

EXERCISE/ACTIVITY
_____
_____
_____
_____
_____

NOTES
_____
_____

HOW I'M FEELING
☺ 😐 ☹

DATE _____   MO TU WE TH FR SA SU

- - - - - - - -   I SLEPT ____ HOURS LAST NIGHT   - - - - - - - -

TODAY I ATE   _____

BREAKFAST
_____
_____
_____
_____

LUNCH
_____
_____
_____
_____
_____

DINNER
_____
_____
_____
_____
_____

— SNACKS —

_____

TOTAL: CALORIES: [_____]

WATER INTAKE ⌷ ⌷ ⌷ ⌷ ⌷ ⌷ ⌷ __ TOTAL OZ.

EXERCISE/ACTIVITY
_____
_____
_____
_____
_____

NOTES
_____
_____

HOW I'M FEELING

☺ 😐 ☹

DATE _____   MO TU WE TH FR SA SU

- - - - - - - -   I SLEPT ____ HOURS LAST NIGHT   - - - - - - - -

TODAY I ATE _____

BREAKFAST
_____
_____
_____
_____

LUNCH
_____
_____
_____
_____

DINNER
_____
_____
_____
_____

—— SNACKS ——
_____

TOTAL: CALORIES: [_____]

WATER INTAKE ⬜⬜⬜⬜⬜⬜⬜ __ **TOTAL OZ.**

EXERCISE/ACTIVITY
_____
_____
_____
_____

NOTES
_____

HOW I'M FEELING
☺ 😐 ☹

DATE _____   MO TU WE TH FR SA SU

- - - - - - - -   I SLEPT ____ HOURS LAST NIGHT   - - - - - - - -

TODAY I ATE   _____

BREAKFAST
_____

_____

_____

_____

LUNCH
_____

_____

_____

_____

DINNER
_____

_____

_____

_____

TOTAL: CALORIES: [_____]

— SNACKS —

WATER INTAKE ⬚⬚⬚⬚⬚⬚⬚ __ TOTAL OZ.

EXERCISE/ACTIVITY
_____

_____

_____

_____

NOTES
_____

_____

HOW I'M FEELING
☺ 😐 ☹

DATE _____   MO TU WE TH FR SA SU

-------- I SLEPT ____ HOURS LAST NIGHT --------

TODAY I ATE _____

BREAKFAST

_____
_____
_____
_____

LUNCH

_____
_____
_____
_____

DINNER

_____
_____
_____
_____

TOTAL: CALORIES: [_____]

—— SNACKS ——

WATER INTAKE ⎕ ⎕ ⎕ ⎕ ⎕ ⎕ ⎕ __ TOTAL OZ.

EXERCISE/ACTIVITY

_____
_____
_____
_____
_____

NOTES   **HOW I'M FEELING**

_____   ☺ 😐 ☹

DATE _____   MO TU WE TH FR SA SU

- - - - - - - -   I SLEPT ____ HOURS LAST NIGHT   - - - - - - - -

TODAY I ATE _____

BREAKFAST
_____
_____
_____
_____

LUNCH
_____
_____
_____
_____
_____

DINNER
_____
_____
_____
_____
_____

—— SNACKS ——

TOTAL: CALORIES: [_____]

WATER INTAKE ⊔ ⊔ ⊔ ⊔ ⊔ ⊔ ⊔ __ TOTAL OZ.

EXERCISE/ACTIVITY
_____
_____
_____
_____
_____

NOTES
_____

HOW I'M FEELING
☺ 😐 ☹

DATE _____   MO TU WE TH FR SA SU

- - - - - - - -   I SLEPT ____ HOURS LAST NIGHT   - - - - - - - -

TODAY I ATE _____

BREAKFAST
_____
_____
_____
_____

— SNACKS —
_____

LUNCH
_____
_____
_____
_____

DINNER
_____
_____
_____
_____

TOTAL: CALORIES: [_____]

WATER INTAKE ⊓ ⊓ ⊓ ⊓ ⊓ ⊓ ⊓ __ **TOTAL OZ.**

EXERCISE/ACTIVITY
_____
_____
_____
_____
_____

NOTES   **HOW I'M FEELING**
_____   ☺ 😐 ☹

DATE _____   MO   TU   WE   TH   FR   SA   SU

- - - - - - - -   **I SLEPT ____ HOURS LAST NIGHT**   - - - - - - - -

TODAY I ATE _____

BREAKFAST

_____

_____

_____

LUNCH

_____

_____

_____

_____

DINNER

_____

_____

_____

_____

TOTAL: CALORIES: [_____]

—— **SNACKS** ——

_____

WATER INTAKE ⎕ ⎕ ⎕ ⎕ ⎕ ⎕ ⎕   __ **TOTAL OZ.**

EXERCISE/ACTIVITY

_____

_____

_____

_____

NOTES   **HOW I'M FEELING**

_____   ☺   😐   ☹

_____

DATE _____ MO TU WE TH FR SA SU

- - - - - - - - I SLEPT ____ HOURS LAST NIGHT - - - - - - - -

TODAY I ATE _____

BREAKFAST

_____
_____
_____
_____

LUNCH

_____
_____
_____
_____

DINNER

_____
_____
_____
_____

TOTAL: CALORIES: [_____]

—— SNACKS ——

_____

WATER INTAKE ⊔ ⊔ ⊔ ⊔ ⊔ ⊔ ⊔ __ **TOTAL OZ.**

EXERCISE/ACTIVITY

_____
_____
_____
_____
_____

NOTES

_____
_____

HOW I'M FEELING

☺ 😐 ☹

DATE _____   MO TU WE TH FR SA SU

| - - - - - - - -   I SLEPT ____ HOURS LAST NIGHT   - - - - - - - - |

TODAY I ATE _____

BREAKFAST
_____
_____
_____
_____

┌─────────────────┐
│ ── SNACKS ──   │
│   │
│   │

LUNCH
_____
_____
_____
_____

DINNER
_____
_____
_____
_____

│   │
│   │
│   │
│ _____ │
└─────────────────┘

TOTAL: CALORIES: [_____]

| WATER INTAKE ⊔ ⊔ ⊔ ⊔ ⊔ ⊔ ⊔ __ TOTAL OZ. |

EXERCISE/ACTIVITY
_____
_____
_____
_____

NOTES   **HOW I'M FEELING**
_____   ☺ 😐 ☹
_____

DATE _____   MO TU WE TH FR SA SU

- - - - - - - -   I SLEPT ____ HOURS LAST NIGHT   - - - - - - - -

TODAY I ATE _____

BREAKFAST

_____
_____
_____
_____

LUNCH

_____
_____
_____
_____

DINNER

_____
_____
_____
_____

TOTAL: CALORIES: [_____]

—— **SNACKS** ——

_____

WATER INTAKE ⊔ ⊔ ⊔ ⊔ ⊔ ⊔ ⊔ __ **TOTAL OZ.**

EXERCISE/ACTIVITY

_____
_____
_____
_____

NOTES   **HOW I'M FEELING**

_____   ☺ 😐 ☹
_____

DATE _____   MO TU WE TH FR SA SU

- - - - - - - -   I SLEPT ____ HOURS LAST NIGHT   - - - - - - - -

TODAY I ATE _____

BREAKFAST
_____
_____
_____
_____

LUNCH
_____
_____
_____
_____

DINNER
_____
_____
_____
_____

— SNACKS —
_____

TOTAL: CALORIES: [_____]

WATER INTAKE ⊔ ⊔ ⊔ ⊔ ⊔ ⊔ ⊔ __ TOTAL OZ.

EXERCISE/ACTIVITY
_____
_____
_____
_____

NOTES   HOW I'M FEELING
_____
_____   ☺ 😐 ☹

DATE _____   MO TU WE TH FR SA SU

- - - - - - - - -   **I SLEPT ____ HOURS LAST NIGHT**   - - - - - - - -

TODAY I ATE _____

BREAKFAST
_____
_____
_____
_____

LUNCH
_____
_____
_____
_____

DINNER
_____
_____
_____
_____

TOTAL: CALORIES: [_____]

—— **SNACKS** ——

WATER INTAKE 🥛🥛🥛🥛🥛🥛🥛 __ **TOTAL OZ.**

EXERCISE/ACTIVITY
_____
_____
_____
_____

NOTES   **HOW I'M FEELING**
_____   ☺ 😐 ☹
_____

DATE _____   MO TU WE TH FR SA SU

- - - - - - - -   I SLEPT ____ HOURS LAST NIGHT   - - - - - - - -

TODAY I ATE _____

BREAKFAST
_____
_____
_____

LUNCH
_____
_____
_____
_____

DINNER
_____
_____
_____
_____

TOTAL: CALORIES: [_____]

—— SNACKS ——

WATER INTAKE ⊔ ⊔ ⊔ ⊔ ⊔ ⊔ ⊔ __ TOTAL OZ.

EXERCISE/ACTIVITY
_____
_____
_____
_____
_____

NOTES   **HOW I'M FEELING**
_____   ☺ 😐 ☹
_____

DATE _____ MO TU WE TH FR SA SU

- - - - - - - -   I SLEPT ____ HOURS LAST NIGHT   - - - - - - - -

TODAY I ATE _____

BREAKFAST
_____

_____

_____

_____

LUNCH
_____

_____

_____

_____

DINNER
_____

_____

_____

_____

TOTAL: CALORIES: [_____]

— SNACKS —

_____

WATER INTAKE 🥛🥛🥛🥛🥛🥛🥛 __ TOTAL OZ.

EXERCISE/ACTIVITY
_____

_____

_____

_____

NOTES
_____

_____

HOW I'M FEELING

☺ 😐 ☹

DATE _____ MO TU WE TH FR SA SU

- - - - - - - -   **I SLEPT ____ HOURS LAST NIGHT**   - - - - - - - -

TODAY I ATE _____

BREAKFAST
_____
_____
_____

LUNCH
_____
_____
_____
_____

DINNER
_____
_____
_____
_____

TOTAL: CALORIES: [_____]

—— **SNACKS** ——

_____

WATER INTAKE 🥛🥛🥛🥛🥛🥛🥛 __ **TOTAL OZ.**

EXERCISE/ACTIVITY
_____
_____
_____
_____

NOTES   **HOW I'M FEELING**
_____   🙂 😐 🙁
_____

DATE _____   MO TU WE TH FR SA SU

- - - - - - - -   I SLEPT ____ HOURS LAST NIGHT   - - - - - - - -

TODAY I ATE _____

BREAKFAST
_____

_____

_____

_____

LUNCH
_____

_____

_____

_____

DINNER
_____

_____

_____

_____

TOTAL: CALORIES: [_____]

— SNACKS —

WATER INTAKE 🥛🥛🥛🥛🥛🥛🥛 __ **TOTAL OZ.**

EXERCISE/ACTIVITY
_____

_____

_____

_____

NOTES   **HOW I'M FEELING**
_____   ☺ 😐 ☹
_____

DATE _____   MO TU WE TH FR SA SU

- - - - - - - -   **I SLEPT ____ HOURS LAST NIGHT**   - - - - - - - -

TODAY I ATE   _____

BREAKFAST
_____
_____
_____
_____

LUNCH
_____
_____
_____
_____

DINNER
_____
_____
_____
_____

—— SNACKS ——

TOTAL: CALORIES: [_____]

WATER INTAKE ⊔ ⊔ ⊔ ⊔ ⊔ ⊔ ⊔ __ **TOTAL OZ.**

EXERCISE/ACTIVITY
_____
_____
_____
_____

NOTES   **HOW I'M FEELING**
_____
_____   ☺ 😐 ☹

DATE _____ MO TU WE TH FR SA SU

- - - - - - - - I SLEPT ____ HOURS LAST NIGHT - - - - - - - -

TODAY I ATE _____

BREAKFAST
_____
_____
_____
_____

LUNCH
_____
_____
_____
_____

DINNER
_____
_____
_____
_____

TOTAL: CALORIES: [_____]

—— SNACKS ——

WATER INTAKE ⨅⨅⨅⨅⨅⨅⨅ __ TOTAL OZ.

EXERCISE/ACTIVITY
_____
_____
_____
_____

NOTES
_____
_____

HOW I'M FEELING

☺ 😐 ☹

DATE _____   MO TU WE TH FR SA SU

- - - - - - - -   I SLEPT ____ HOURS LAST NIGHT   - - - - - - - -

TODAY I ATE _____

BREAKFAST
_____
_____
_____
_____

LUNCH
_____
_____
_____
_____
_____

DINNER
_____
_____
_____
_____

TOTAL: CALORIES: [_____]

—— SNACKS ——

WATER INTAKE ⊔ ⊔ ⊔ ⊔ ⊔ ⊔ ⊔ __ TOTAL OZ.

EXERCISE/ACTIVITY
_____
_____
_____
_____

NOTES
_____

HOW I'M FEELING
☺ 😐 ☹

DATE _____   MO TU WE TH FR SA SU

- - - - - - - -   I SLEPT ____ HOURS LAST NIGHT   - - - - - - - -

TODAY I ATE _____

BREAKFAST
_____
_____
_____
_____

LUNCH
_____
_____
_____
_____

DINNER
_____
_____
_____
_____

TOTAL: CALORIES: [_____]

—— SNACKS ——

_____

WATER INTAKE ⬜⬜⬜⬜⬜⬜⬜ __ TOTAL OZ.

EXERCISE/ACTIVITY
_____
_____
_____
_____
_____

NOTES
_____

HOW I'M FEELING
☺ 😐 ☹

DATE _____   MO   TU   WE   TH   FR   SA   SU

- - - - - - - -   I SLEPT _____ HOURS LAST NIGHT   - - - - - - - -

TODAY I ATE _____

BREAKFAST
_____
_____
_____
_____

LUNCH
_____
_____
_____
_____

DINNER
_____
_____
_____
_____

— SNACKS —

TOTAL: CALORIES: [_____]

WATER INTAKE ☐ ☐ ☐ ☐ ☐ ☐ ☐ __ TOTAL OZ.

EXERCISE/ACTIVITY
_____
_____
_____
_____

NOTES
_____
_____

HOW I'M FEELING
☺   😐   ☹

DATE _____   MO   TU   WE   TH   FR   SA   SU

> - - - - - - - -   I SLEPT ____ HOURS LAST NIGHT   - - - - - - - -

TODAY I ATE _____

BREAKFAST

_____

_____

_____

_____

LUNCH

_____

_____

_____

_____

DINNER

_____

_____

_____

_____

TOTAL: CALORIES: [_____]

— SNACKS —

_____

WATER INTAKE ⊔⊔⊔⊔⊔⊔⊔ __ TOTAL OZ.

EXERCISE/ACTIVITY

_____

_____

_____

_____

_____

NOTES   **HOW I'M FEELING**

_____   ☺   ☺   ☹

DATE _____   MO TU WE TH FR SA SU

- - - - - - - -   **I SLEPT** ____ **HOURS LAST NIGHT**   - - - - - - - -

TODAY I ATE   _____

BREAKFAST

_____
_____
_____
_____

LUNCH

_____
_____
_____
_____

DINNER

_____
_____
_____
_____

TOTAL: CALORIES: [_____]

—— **SNACKS** ——

WATER INTAKE ⑃⑃⑃⑃⑃⑃⑃ __ **TOTAL OZ.**

EXERCISE/ACTIVITY

_____
_____
_____
_____
_____

NOTES   **HOW I'M FEELING**

_____
_____   ☺ 😐 ☹

DATE _____   MO TU WE TH FR SA SU

- - - - - - - -   I SLEPT ____ HOURS LAST NIGHT   - - - - - - - -

TODAY I ATE _____

BREAKFAST
_____
_____
_____
_____

LUNCH
_____
_____
_____
_____

DINNER
_____
_____
_____
_____

TOTAL: CALORIES: [_____]

— SNACKS —

WATER INTAKE ⊓ ⊓ ⊓ ⊓ ⊓ ⊓ ⊓ __ TOTAL OZ.

EXERCISE/ACTIVITY
_____
_____
_____
_____

NOTES
_____
_____

HOW I'M FEELING
☺ 😐 ☹

DATE _____   MO TU WE TH FR SA SU

- - - - - - - -   I SLEPT ____ HOURS LAST NIGHT   - - - - - - - -

TODAY I ATE _____

BREAKFAST
_____
_____
_____
_____

LUNCH
_____
_____
_____
_____

DINNER
_____
_____
_____
_____

TOTAL: CALORIES: [_____]

—— SNACKS ——

WATER INTAKE [glass][glass][glass][glass][glass][glass][glass] __ TOTAL OZ.

EXERCISE/ACTIVITY
_____
_____
_____
_____
_____

NOTES   **HOW I'M FEELING**
_____
_____   :)   :| :(

DATE _____   MO TU WE TH FR SA SU

- - - - - - - -   I SLEPT ____ HOURS LAST NIGHT   - - - - - - - -

TODAY I ATE _____

BREAKFAST
_____
_____
_____
_____

LUNCH
_____
_____
_____
_____

DINNER
_____
_____
_____
_____

TOTAL: CALORIES: [_____]

— SNACKS —

_____

WATER INTAKE ⬚⬚⬚⬚⬚⬚⬚ __ TOTAL OZ.

EXERCISE/ACTIVITY
_____
_____
_____
_____

NOTES   **HOW I'M FEELING**
_____   ☺ 😐 ☹
_____

DATE _____   MO TU WE TH FR SA SU

- - - - - - - -   I SLEPT ____ HOURS LAST NIGHT   - - - - - - - -

TODAY I ATE   _____

BREAKFAST
_____
_____
_____
_____

LUNCH
_____
_____
_____
_____

DINNER
_____
_____
_____
_____

—— SNACKS ——

TOTAL: CALORIES: [   ]

WATER INTAKE ⊔ ⊔ ⊔ ⊔ ⊔ ⊔ ⊔ __ TOTAL OZ.

EXERCISE/ACTIVITY
_____
_____
_____
_____

NOTES   HOW I'M FEELING
_____   ☺ 😐 ☹
_____

DATE _____ MO TU WE TH FR SA SU

- - - - - - - -   I SLEPT ____ HOURS LAST NIGHT   - - - - - - - -

TODAY I ATE _____

BREAKFAST
_____
_____
_____
_____

LUNCH
_____
_____
_____
_____

DINNER
_____
_____
_____
_____

TOTAL: CALORIES: [_____]

—— SNACKS ——
_____

WATER INTAKE ⊓⊓⊓⊓⊓⊓⊓ __ TOTAL OZ.

EXERCISE/ACTIVITY
_____
_____
_____
_____

NOTES
_____
_____

HOW I'M FEELING
☺ 😐 ☹

DATE _____ MO TU WE TH FR SA SU

- - - - - - - - I SLEPT ____ HOURS LAST NIGHT - - - - - - - -

TODAY I ATE _____

BREAKFAST

_____
_____
_____
_____

LUNCH

_____
_____
_____
_____

DINNER

_____
_____
_____
_____

—— SNACKS ——

TOTAL: CALORIES: \[_____\]

WATER INTAKE ⊔ ⊔ ⊔ ⊔ ⊔ ⊔ ⊔ __ TOTAL OZ.

EXERCISE/ACTIVITY

_____
_____
_____
_____

NOTES   **HOW I'M FEELING**

_____   ☺ ☺ ☹
_____

DATE _____   MO TU WE TH FR SA SU

- - - - - - - -   I SLEPT ____ HOURS LAST NIGHT   - - - - - - - -

TODAY I ATE _____

BREAKFAST
_____
_____
_____
_____

LUNCH
_____
_____
_____
_____

DINNER
_____
_____
_____
_____

TOTAL: CALORIES: [_____]

—— **SNACKS** ——
_____

WATER INTAKE ⎕⎕⎕⎕⎕⎕⎕ __ **TOTAL OZ.**

EXERCISE/ACTIVITY
_____
_____
_____
_____
_____

NOTES   **HOW I'M FEELING**
_____ ☺ ☺ ☹

DATE _____   MO TU WE TH FR SA SU

- - - - - - - -   I SLEPT ____ HOURS LAST NIGHT   - - - - - - - -

TODAY I ATE _____

BREAKFAST
_____
_____
_____
_____

LUNCH
_____
_____
_____
_____

DINNER
_____
_____
_____
_____

TOTAL: CALORIES: [_____]

—— SNACKS ——

WATER INTAKE ⊔ ⊔ ⊔ ⊔ ⊔ ⊔ ⊔ __ TOTAL OZ.

EXERCISE/ACTIVITY
_____
_____
_____
_____

NOTES   **HOW I'M FEELING**
_____
_____   ☺ 😐 ☹

DATE _____ MO TU WE TH FR SA SU

- - - - - - - - I SLEPT ____ HOURS LAST NIGHT - - - - - - - -

TODAY I ATE _____

BREAKFAST

_____

_____

_____

_____

LUNCH

_____

_____

_____

_____

DINNER

_____

_____

_____

_____

TOTAL: CALORIES: [_____]

— SNACKS —

WATER INTAKE ⬛⬛⬛⬛⬛⬛⬛ __ TOTAL OZ.

EXERCISE/ACTIVITY

_____

_____

_____

_____

NOTES

_____

HOW I'M FEELING

☺ 😐 ☹

DATE _____ MO TU WE TH FR SA SU

- - - - - - - - **I SLEPT ____ HOURS LAST NIGHT** - - - - - - - -

TODAY I ATE _____

BREAKFAST
_____
_____
_____
_____

LUNCH
_____
_____
_____
_____

DINNER
_____
_____
_____
_____

TOTAL: CALORIES: [_____]

—— **SNACKS** ——

WATER INTAKE ⬜⬜⬜⬜⬜⬜⬜ __ **TOTAL OZ.**

EXERCISE/ACTIVITY
_____
_____
_____
_____
_____

NOTES   **HOW I'M FEELING**
_____   ☺ ☺ ☹
_____

DATE _____ MO TU WE TH FR SA SU

-------- **I SLEPT ____ HOURS LAST NIGHT** --------

TODAY I ATE _____

BREAKFAST

_____

_____

_____

_____

— SNACKS —

LUNCH

_____

_____

_____

_____

DINNER

_____

_____

_____

_____

_____

TOTAL: CALORIES: [_____]

WATER INTAKE ⊔⊔⊔⊔⊔⊔⊔ __ **TOTAL OZ.**

EXERCISE/ACTIVITY

_____

_____

_____

_____

NOTES

_____

_____

HOW I'M FEELING

☺ ☺ ☹

DATE _____   MO   TU   WE   TH   FR   SA   SU

- - - - - - - -   **I SLEPT ____ HOURS LAST NIGHT**   - - - - - - - -

TODAY I ATE _____

BREAKFAST

_____

_____

_____

_____

LUNCH

_____

_____

_____

_____

DINNER

_____

_____

_____

_____

TOTAL: CALORIES: [_____]

—— **SNACKS** ——

WATER INTAKE   ⬜ ⬜ ⬜ ⬜ ⬜ ⬜ ⬜   __ **TOTAL OZ.**

EXERCISE/ACTIVITY

_____

_____

_____

_____

NOTES   **HOW I'M FEELING**

_____

_____   ☺   😐   ☹

DATE _____ MO TU WE TH FR SA SU

- - - - - - - I SLEPT ____ HOURS LAST NIGHT - - - - - - - -

TODAY I ATE _____

BREAKFAST
_____
_____
_____
_____

LUNCH
_____
_____
_____
_____

DINNER
_____
_____
_____
_____

TOTAL: CALORIES: [_____]

--- SNACKS ---

_____

WATER INTAKE ⬜ ⬜ ⬜ ⬜ ⬜ ⬜ ⬜ __ TOTAL OZ.

EXERCISE/ACTIVITY
_____
_____
_____
_____

NOTES
_____

HOW I'M FEELING
☺ 😐 ☹

DATE _____   MO   TU   WE   TH   FR   SA   SU

- - - - - - - -   **I SLEPT** ____ **HOURS LAST NIGHT**   - - - - - - - -

TODAY I ATE _____

BREAKFAST

_____
_____
_____
_____

LUNCH

_____
_____
_____
_____

DINNER

_____
_____
_____
_____

—— **SNACKS** ——

TOTAL: CALORIES: [_____]

WATER INTAKE 🥛🥛🥛🥛🥛🥛🥛 __ **TOTAL OZ.**

EXERCISE/ACTIVITY

_____
_____
_____
_____
_____

NOTES

_____

HOW I'M FEELING

☺   😐   ☹

DATE _____ MO TU WE TH FR SA SU

- - - - - - - - I SLEPT ____ HOURS LAST NIGHT - - - - - - - -

TODAY I ATE _____

BREAKFAST

_____

_____

_____

_____

LUNCH

_____

_____

_____

_____

DINNER

_____

_____

_____

_____

TOTAL: CALORIES: [_____]

— SNACKS —

_____

WATER INTAKE ⬜⬜⬜⬜⬜⬜⬜ __ TOTAL OZ.

EXERCISE/ACTIVITY

_____

_____

_____

_____

NOTES

_____

HOW I'M FEELING

☺ 😐 ☹

DATE _____ MO TU WE TH FR SA SU

- - - - - - - -   **I SLEPT ____ HOURS LAST NIGHT**   - - - - - - - -

TODAY I ATE _____

BREAKFAST

_____
_____
_____
_____

LUNCH

_____
_____
_____
_____

DINNER

_____
_____
_____
_____

SNACKS

TOTAL: CALORIES: [_____]

WATER INTAKE ⬜⬜⬜⬜⬜⬜⬜ __ **TOTAL OZ.**

EXERCISE/ACTIVITY

_____
_____
_____
_____

NOTES   **HOW I'M FEELING**

_____   ☺ 😐 ☹
_____

DATE _____ MO TU WE TH FR SA SU

- - - - - - - - I SLEPT ____ HOURS LAST NIGHT - - - - - - - -

TODAY I ATE _____

BREAKFAST

_____

_____

_____

_____

LUNCH

_____

_____

_____

_____

DINNER

_____

_____

_____

_____

TOTAL: CALORIES: [_____]

—— SNACKS ——

_____

WATER INTAKE ⊔⊔⊔⊔⊔⊔⊔ __ TOTAL OZ.

EXERCISE/ACTIVITY

_____

_____

_____

_____

NOTES

_____

_____

HOW I'M FEELING

☺ 😐 ☹

DATE _____   MO TU WE TH FR SA SU

- - - - - - - -   I SLEPT ____ HOURS LAST NIGHT   - - - - - - - -

TODAY I ATE _____

BREAKFAST
_____
_____
_____
_____

LUNCH
_____
_____
_____
_____

DINNER
_____
_____
_____
_____

— SNACKS —

TOTAL: CALORIES: [_____]

WATER INTAKE 🥛🥛🥛🥛🥛🥛🥛 __ TOTAL OZ.

EXERCISE/ACTIVITY
_____
_____
_____
_____

NOTES   **HOW I'M FEELING**
_____
_____   ☺ 😐 ☹

DATE _____   MO TU WE TH FR SA SU

- - - - - - - - I SLEPT ____ HOURS LAST NIGHT - - - - - - - -

TODAY I ATE _____

BREAKFAST
_____
_____
_____
_____

LUNCH
_____
_____
_____
_____

DINNER
_____
_____
_____
_____

TOTAL: CALORIES: [_____]

— SNACKS —

WATER INTAKE ⊔⊔⊔⊔⊔⊔⊔ __ TOTAL OZ.

EXERCISE/ACTIVITY
_____
_____
_____
_____

NOTES   **HOW I'M FEELING**
_____
_____   ☺ 😐 ☹

DATE _____ MO TU WE TH FR SA SU

-------- **I SLEPT ____ HOURS LAST NIGHT** --------

TODAY I ATE _____

BREAKFAST
_____
_____
_____

LUNCH
_____
_____
_____
_____

DINNER
_____
_____
_____
_____

TOTAL: CALORIES: [_____]

—— **SNACKS** ——

WATER INTAKE 🥛🥛🥛🥛🥛🥛🥛 __ **TOTAL OZ.**

EXERCISE/ACTIVITY
_____
_____
_____
_____

NOTES
_____

HOW I'M FEELING

☺ 😐 ☹

DATE _____   MO TU WE TH FR SA SU

- - - - - - - -   I SLEPT ____ HOURS LAST NIGHT   - - - - - - - -

TODAY I ATE _____

BREAKFAST
_____
_____
_____
_____

LUNCH
_____
_____
_____
_____

DINNER
_____
_____
_____
_____

— SNACKS —
_____

TOTAL: CALORIES: [_____]

WATER INTAKE ⊔⊔⊔⊔⊔⊔⊔ __ TOTAL OZ.

EXERCISE/ACTIVITY
_____
_____
_____
_____

NOTES
_____

HOW I'M FEELING
☺ ☺ ☹

DATE _____   MO TU WE TH FR SA SU

- - - - - - - -   I SLEPT ____ HOURS LAST NIGHT   - - - - - - - -

TODAY I ATE   _____

BREAKFAST
_____
_____
_____
_____

LUNCH
_____
_____
_____
_____

DINNER
_____
_____
_____
_____

TOTAL: CALORIES: [_____]

—— **SNACKS** ——

WATER INTAKE ⬜⬜⬜⬜⬜⬜⬜ __ **TOTAL OZ.**

EXERCISE/ACTIVITY
_____
_____
_____
_____
_____

NOTES   **HOW I'M FEELING**
_____
_____   ☺ 😐 ☹

DATE _____   MO TU WE TH FR SA SU

- - - - - - - -   I SLEPT ____ HOURS LAST NIGHT   - - - - - - - -

TODAY I ATE _____

BREAKFAST
_____
_____
_____
_____

LUNCH
_____
_____
_____
_____

DINNER
_____
_____
_____
_____

— SNACKS —

_____

TOTAL: CALORIES: [_____]

WATER INTAKE ⊔⊔⊔⊔⊔⊔⊔ __ **TOTAL OZ.**

EXERCISE/ACTIVITY
_____
_____
_____
_____

NOTES
_____
_____

HOW I'M FEELING

☺ 😐 ☹

DATE _____ MO TU WE TH FR SA SU

- - - - - - - - **I SLEPT ____ HOURS LAST NIGHT** - - - - - - - -

TODAY I ATE _____

BREAKFAST
_____
_____
_____
_____

LUNCH
_____
_____
_____
_____

DINNER
_____
_____
_____
_____

—— **SNACKS** ——

TOTAL: CALORIES: [_____]

WATER INTAKE ⊔ ⊔ ⊔ ⊔ ⊔ ⊔ ⊔ __ **TOTAL OZ.**

EXERCISE/ACTIVITY
_____
_____
_____
_____
_____

NOTES
_____

HOW I'M FEELING

☺ 😐 ☹

DATE _____   MO TU WE TH FR SA SU

- - - - - - - -   I SLEPT ____ HOURS LAST NIGHT   - - - - - - - -

TODAY I ATE _____

BREAKFAST

_____

_____

_____

_____

LUNCH

_____

_____

_____

_____

DINNER

_____

_____

_____

_____

TOTAL: CALORIES: [_____]

— SNACKS —

_____

WATER INTAKE 🥛🥛🥛🥛🥛🥛🥛 __ TOTAL OZ.

EXERCISE/ACTIVITY

_____

_____

_____

_____

_____

NOTES   **HOW I'M FEELING**

_____   ☺ 😐 ☹

_____

DATE _____   MO TU WE TH FR SA SU

- - - - - - - -   **I SLEPT ____ HOURS LAST NIGHT**   - - - - - - - -

TODAY I ATE _____

BREAKFAST
_____

_____

_____

_____

LUNCH
_____

_____

_____

_____

DINNER
_____

_____

_____

_____

TOTAL: CALORIES: [_____]

—— **SNACKS** ——

WATER INTAKE 🥛🥛🥛🥛🥛🥛🥛 __ **TOTAL OZ.**

EXERCISE/ACTIVITY
_____

_____

_____

_____

_____

NOTES   **HOW I'M FEELING**
_____   ☺ 😐 ☹
_____

DATE _____   MO TU WE TH FR SA SU

- - - - - - - -   I SLEPT ____ HOURS LAST NIGHT   - - - - - - - -

TODAY I ATE _____

BREAKFAST
_____
_____
_____
_____

LUNCH
_____
_____
_____
_____

DINNER
_____
_____
_____
_____

TOTAL: CALORIES: [_____]

— SNACKS —
_____

WATER INTAKE ⊔ ⊔ ⊔ ⊔ ⊔ ⊔ ⊔ __ TOTAL OZ.

EXERCISE/ACTIVITY
_____
_____
_____
_____

NOTES
_____
_____

HOW I'M FEELING
☺ 😐 ☹

DATE _____   MO   TU   WE   TH   FR   SA   SU

--------   I SLEPT ____ HOURS LAST NIGHT   --------

TODAY I ATE _____

BREAKFAST
_____
_____
_____
_____

LUNCH
_____
_____
_____
_____

DINNER
_____
_____
_____
_____

TOTAL: CALORIES: [_____]

—— **SNACKS** ——

WATER INTAKE ⬜⬜⬜⬜⬜⬜⬜ __ **TOTAL OZ.**

EXERCISE/ACTIVITY
_____
_____
_____
_____
_____

NOTES   **HOW I'M FEELING**
_____   ☺ 😐 ☹
_____

DATE _____   MO TU WE TH FR SA SU

- - - - - - - -   I SLEPT ____ HOURS LAST NIGHT   - - - - - - - -

TODAY I ATE _____

BREAKFAST

_____

_____

_____

_____

LUNCH

_____

_____

_____

_____

DINNER

_____

_____

_____

_____

TOTAL: CALORIES: [_____]

— SNACKS —

_____

WATER INTAKE 🥛🥛🥛🥛🥛🥛🥛 __ TOTAL OZ.

EXERCISE/ACTIVITY

_____

_____

_____

_____

_____

NOTES

_____

HOW I'M FEELING

☺ 😐 ☹

DATE _____   MO TU WE TH FR SA SU

- - - - - - - -   **I SLEPT ____ HOURS LAST NIGHT**   - - - - - - - -

TODAY I ATE _____

BREAKFAST

_____

_____

_____

_____

LUNCH

_____

_____

_____

_____

DINNER

_____

_____

_____

_____

TOTAL: CALORIES: [_____]

—— **SNACKS** ——

_____

WATER INTAKE ⊔ ⊔ ⊔ ⊔ ⊔ ⊔ ⊔ __ **TOTAL OZ.**

EXERCISE/ACTIVITY

_____

_____

_____

_____

_____

NOTES   **HOW I'M FEELING**

_____   ☺ 😐 ☹

_____

DATE _____   MO   TU   WE   TH   FR   SA   SU

- - - - - - - -   **I SLEPT** ____ **HOURS LAST NIGHT**   - - - - - - - -

TODAY I ATE _____

BREAKFAST
_____
_____
_____
_____

LUNCH
_____
_____
_____
_____

DINNER
_____
_____
_____
_____

TOTAL: CALORIES: [_____]

┌─ **SNACKS** ─┐

_____

WATER INTAKE 🥛🥛🥛🥛🥛🥛🥛 __ **TOTAL OZ.**

EXERCISE/ACTIVITY
_____
_____
_____
_____

NOTES   **HOW I'M FEELING**
_____   ☺ ☺ ☹
_____

DATE _____ MO TU WE TH FR SA SU

- - - - - - - - **I SLEPT ____ HOURS LAST NIGHT** - - - - - - - -

TODAY I ATE _____

BREAKFAST
_____
_____
_____
_____

LUNCH
_____
_____
_____
_____

DINNER
_____
_____
_____
_____

TOTAL: CALORIES: _____

—— **SNACKS** ——

WATER INTAKE ⊔ ⊔ ⊔ ⊔ ⊔ ⊔ ⊔ __ **TOTAL OZ.**

EXERCISE/ACTIVITY
_____
_____
_____
_____
_____

NOTES
_____
_____

HOW I'M FEELING
☺ 😐 ☹

DATE _____   MO TU WE TH FR SA SU

- - - - - - - -   I SLEPT ____ HOURS LAST NIGHT   - - - - - - - -

TODAY I ATE _____

BREAKFAST
_____
_____
_____
_____

LUNCH
_____
_____
_____
_____

DINNER
_____
_____
_____
_____

TOTAL: CALORIES: [_____]

— SNACKS —

WATER INTAKE 🥛🥛🥛🥛🥛🥛🥛 __ TOTAL OZ.

EXERCISE/ACTIVITY
_____
_____
_____
_____

NOTES   **HOW I'M FEELING**
_____   ☺ 😐 ☹
_____

DATE _____   MO TU WE TH FR SA SU

- - - - - - - -   I SLEPT ____ HOURS LAST NIGHT   - - - - - - - -

TODAY I ATE _____

BREAKFAST
_____
_____
_____
_____

LUNCH
_____
_____
_____
_____

DINNER
_____
_____
_____
_____

TOTAL: CALORIES: [_____]

—— SNACKS ——

WATER INTAKE ⬛⬛⬛⬛⬛⬛⬛ __ TOTAL OZ.

EXERCISE/ACTIVITY
_____
_____
_____
_____
_____

NOTES   HOW I'M FEELING
_____   ☺ 😐 ☹
_____

DATE _____ MO TU WE TH FR SA SU

- - - - - - - - I SLEPT ____ HOURS LAST NIGHT - - - - - - - -

TODAY I ATE _____

BREAKFAST
_____
_____
_____
_____

LUNCH
_____
_____
_____
_____

DINNER
_____
_____
_____
_____

TOTAL: CALORIES: [_____]

—— SNACKS ——

_____

WATER INTAKE 🥤🥤🥤🥤🥤🥤🥤 __ TOTAL OZ.

EXERCISE/ACTIVITY
_____
_____
_____
_____
_____

NOTES   HOW I'M FEELING
_____
_____   ☺ 😐 ☹

DATE _____   MO TU WE TH FR SA SU

| - - - - - - - -   I SLEPT ____ HOURS LAST NIGHT   - - - - - - - - |

TODAY I ATE _____

BREAKFAST
_____
_____
_____
_____

LUNCH
_____
_____
_____
_____

DINNER
_____
_____
_____
_____

TOTAL: CALORIES: [_____]

—— **SNACKS** ——

_____

WATER INTAKE 🥛🥛🥛🥛🥛🥛🥛 __ **TOTAL OZ.**

EXERCISE/ACTIVITY
_____
_____
_____
_____
_____

NOTES   **HOW I'M FEELING**
_____   ☺ 😐 ☹

DATE _____   MO TU WE TH FR SA SU

- - - - - - - -   I SLEPT ____ HOURS LAST NIGHT   - - - - - - - -

TODAY I ATE _____

BREAKFAST
_____
_____
_____
_____

LUNCH
_____
_____
_____
_____

DINNER
_____
_____
_____
_____

TOTAL: CALORIES: [_____]

—— SNACKS ——

_____

WATER INTAKE ⊔ ⊔ ⊔ ⊔ ⊔ ⊔ ⊔ __ TOTAL OZ.

EXERCISE/ACTIVITY
_____
_____
_____
_____
_____

NOTES
_____
_____

HOW I'M FEELING

☺ 😐 ☹

DATE _____   MO TU WE TH FR SA SU

- - - - - - - -   I SLEPT ____ HOURS LAST NIGHT   - - - - - - - -

TODAY I ATE _____

BREAKFAST

_____

_____

_____

_____

LUNCH

_____

_____

_____

_____

DINNER

_____

_____

_____

_____

TOTAL: CALORIES: [_____]

— SNACKS —

WATER INTAKE ⬜⬜⬜⬜⬜⬜⬜ __ TOTAL OZ.

EXERCISE/ACTIVITY

_____

_____

_____

_____

_____

NOTES   **HOW I'M FEELING**

_____   ☺ ☺ ☹

_____

DATE _____   MO TU WE TH FR SA SU

- - - - - - - -   **I SLEPT ____ HOURS LAST NIGHT**   - - - - - - - -

TODAY I ATE _____

BREAKFAST
_____
_____
_____
_____

LUNCH
_____
_____
_____
_____

DINNER
_____
_____
_____
_____

TOTAL: CALORIES: [_____]

— SNACKS —

_____

WATER INTAKE ⬚⬚⬚⬚⬚⬚ __ **TOTAL OZ.**

EXERCISE/ACTIVITY
_____
_____
_____
_____

NOTES
_____
_____

HOW I'M FEELING

☺ 😐 ☹

DATE _____   MO TU WE TH FR SA SU

- - - - - - - -   I SLEPT ____ HOURS LAST NIGHT   - - - - - - - -

TODAY I ATE _____

BREAKFAST

_____

_____

_____

_____

LUNCH

_____

_____

_____

_____

DINNER

_____

_____

_____

_____

TOTAL: CALORIES: [_____]

—— **SNACKS** ——

WATER INTAKE 🥛🥛🥛🥛🥛🥛🥛 ___ **TOTAL OZ.**

EXERCISE/ACTIVITY

_____

_____

_____

_____

_____

NOTES   **HOW I'M FEELING**

_____   ☺ 😐 ☹

_____

DATE _____ MO TU WE TH FR SA SU

- - - - - - - - I SLEPT ____ HOURS LAST NIGHT - - - - - - - -

TODAY I ATE _____

BREAKFAST

_____
_____
_____
_____

LUNCH

_____
_____
_____
_____

DINNER

_____
_____
_____
_____

TOTAL: CALORIES: [_____]

— SNACKS —

_____

WATER INTAKE ⊔ ⊔ ⊔ ⊔ ⊔ ⊔ ⊔ __ TOTAL OZ.

EXERCISE/ACTIVITY

_____
_____
_____
_____

NOTES

_____
_____

HOW I'M FEELING

☺ 😐 ☹

DATE _____   MO TU WE TH FR SA SU

- - - - - - - -   I SLEPT ____ HOURS LAST NIGHT   - - - - - - - -

TODAY I ATE _____

BREAKFAST
_____
_____
_____

┌──────────────────┐
│ —— SNACKS ——   │
│   │
LUNCH
_____
_____
_____

DINNER
_____
_____
_____
_____

TOTAL: CALORIES: [_____]

WATER INTAKE 🥛🥛🥛🥛🥛🥛🥛 __ **TOTAL OZ.**

EXERCISE/ACTIVITY
_____
_____
_____
_____
_____

NOTES   **HOW I'M FEELING**
_____
_____   ☺ 😐 ☹

DATE _____ MO TU WE TH FR SA SU

- - - - - - - - I SLEPT ____ HOURS LAST NIGHT   - - - - - - - -

TODAY I ATE _____

BREAKFAST

_____
_____
_____
_____

LUNCH

_____
_____
_____
_____

DINNER

_____
_____
_____
_____

— SNACKS —

TOTAL: CALORIES: [_____]

WATER INTAKE ⎕ ⎕ ⎕ ⎕ ⎕ ⎕ ⎕ __ TOTAL OZ.

EXERCISE/ACTIVITY

_____
_____
_____
_____

NOTES   **HOW I'M FEELING**

_____
_____   ☺ 😐 ☹

DATE _____ MO TU WE TH FR SA SU

- - - - - - - - | I SLEPT ____ HOURS LAST NIGHT | - - - - - - - -

TODAY I ATE _____

BREAKFAST
_____
_____
_____
_____

LUNCH
_____
_____
_____
_____

DINNER
_____
_____
_____
_____

TOTAL: CALORIES: [_____]

—— SNACKS ——

WATER INTAKE 🥛🥛🥛🥛🥛🥛🥛 ___ TOTAL OZ.

EXERCISE/ACTIVITY
_____
_____
_____
_____
_____

NOTES
_____

HOW I'M FEELING
🙂 😐 🙁

DATE _____ MO TU WE TH FR SA SU

- - - - - - - - **I SLEPT ____ HOURS LAST NIGHT** - - - - - - - -

TODAY I ATE _____

BREAKFAST

_____

_____

_____

_____

LUNCH

_____

_____

_____

_____

_____

DINNER

_____

_____

_____

_____

_____

TOTAL: CALORIES: [_____]

— **SNACKS** —

_____

WATER INTAKE 🥛🥛🥛🥛🥛🥛🥛 ___ **TOTAL OZ.**

EXERCISE/ACTIVITY

_____

_____

_____

_____

NOTES

_____

_____

HOW I'M FEELING

☺ 😐 ☹

DATE _____   MO TU WE TH FR SA SU

- - - - - - - -   **I SLEPT ____ HOURS LAST NIGHT**   - - - - - - - -

TODAY I ATE _____

BREAKFAST

_____

_____

_____

LUNCH

_____

_____

_____

_____

DINNER

_____

_____

_____

_____

TOTAL: CALORIES: [_____]

— **SNACKS** —

WATER INTAKE ▯ ▯ ▯ ▯ ▯ ▯ ▯ __ **TOTAL OZ.**

EXERCISE/ACTIVITY

_____

_____

_____

_____

_____

NOTES

_____

_____

HOW I'M FEELING

☺ 😐 ☹

DATE _____ MO TU WE TH FR SA SU

- - - - - - - - I SLEPT ____ HOURS LAST NIGHT - - - - - - - -

TODAY I ATE _____

BREAKFAST
_____

_____

_____

_____

LUNCH
_____

_____

_____

_____

DINNER
_____

_____

_____

_____

TOTAL: CALORIES: [_____]

—— SNACKS ——

_____

WATER INTAKE 🥛🥛🥛🥛🥛🥛🥛 __ TOTAL OZ.

EXERCISE/ACTIVITY
_____

_____

_____

_____

_____

NOTES
_____

_____

HOW I'M FEELING

☺ 😐 ☹

DATE _____   MO TU WE TH FR SA SU

- - - - - - - -   **I SLEPT ____ HOURS LAST NIGHT**   - - - - - - - -

TODAY I ATE _____

BREAKFAST

_____

_____

_____

_____

LUNCH

_____

_____

_____

_____

DINNER

_____

_____

_____

_____

TOTAL: CALORIES: [_____]

— **SNACKS** —

_____

WATER INTAKE ⬜⬜⬜⬜⬜⬜⬜ __ **TOTAL OZ.**

EXERCISE/ACTIVITY

_____

_____

_____

_____

_____

NOTES

_____

_____

HOW I'M FEELING

☺ 😐 ☹

DATE _____   MO TU WE TH FR SA SU

- - - - - - - -   I SLEPT ____ HOURS LAST NIGHT   - - - - - - - -

TODAY I ATE _____

BREAKFAST
_____
_____
_____
_____

LUNCH
_____
_____
_____
_____

DINNER
_____
_____
_____
_____

TOTAL: CALORIES: [_____]

—— SNACKS ——

_____

WATER INTAKE ⊔ ⊔ ⊔ ⊔ ⊔ ⊔ ⊔ __ TOTAL OZ.

EXERCISE/ACTIVITY
_____
_____
_____
_____
_____

NOTES
_____
_____

HOW I'M FEELING

☺ ☺ ☹

DATE _____   MO TU WE TH FR SA SU

- - - - - - - - | **I SLEPT ____ HOURS LAST NIGHT** | - - - - - - - -

TODAY I ATE _____

BREAKFAST
_____
_____
_____
_____

LUNCH
_____
_____
_____
_____

DINNER
_____
_____
_____
_____

TOTAL: CALORIES: [_____]

—— **SNACKS** ——

WATER INTAKE ⊔⊔⊔⊔⊔⊔⊔ __ **TOTAL OZ.**

EXERCISE/ACTIVITY
_____
_____
_____
_____
_____

NOTES
_____

HOW I'M FEELING

☺ 😐 ☹

DATE _____   MO   TU   WE   TH   FR   SA   SU

- - - - - - - - I SLEPT ____ HOURS LAST NIGHT - - - - - - - -

TODAY I ATE _____

BREAKFAST

_____

_____

_____

_____

LUNCH

_____

_____

_____

_____

DINNER

_____

_____

_____

_____

TOTAL: CALORIES: [_____]

— SNACKS —

WATER INTAKE   ⊔ ⊔ ⊔ ⊔ ⊔ ⊔ ⊔   __ TOTAL OZ.

EXERCISE/ACTIVITY

_____

_____

_____

_____

NOTES

_____

HOW I'M FEELING

☺   😐   ☹

DATE _____ MO TU WE TH FR SA SU

- - - - - - - -   I SLEPT ____ HOURS LAST NIGHT   - - - - - - - -

TODAY I ATE _____

BREAKFAST
_____
_____
_____
_____

LUNCH
_____
_____
_____
_____

DINNER
_____
_____
_____
_____

TOTAL: CALORIES: [_____]

—— SNACKS ——

WATER INTAKE 🥛🥛🥛🥛🥛🥛🥛 __ TOTAL OZ.

EXERCISE/ACTIVITY
_____
_____
_____
_____
_____

NOTES
_____

HOW I'M FEELING

☺ 😐 ☹

DATE _____ MO TU WE TH FR SA SU

- - - - - - - - I SLEPT ____ HOURS LAST NIGHT - - - - - - - -

TODAY I ATE _____

BREAKFAST

_____
_____
_____
_____

LUNCH

_____
_____
_____
_____

DINNER

_____
_____
_____
_____

TOTAL: CALORIES: [_____]

— SNACKS —

_____

WATER INTAKE 🥛🥛🥛🥛🥛🥛🥛 __ TOTAL OZ.

EXERCISE/ACTIVITY

_____
_____
_____
_____
_____

NOTES   **HOW I'M FEELING**

_____   ☺ 😐 ☹
_____

DATE _____   MO TU WE TH FR SA SU

- - - - - - - -   I SLEPT ____ HOURS LAST NIGHT   - - - - - - - -

TODAY I ATE _____

BREAKFAST

_____

_____

_____

LUNCH

_____

_____

_____

DINNER

_____

_____

_____

_____

— SNACKS —

TOTAL: CALORIES: [_____]

WATER INTAKE ▢ ▢ ▢ ▢ ▢ ▢ ▢ __ TOTAL OZ.

EXERCISE/ACTIVITY

_____

_____

_____

_____

NOTES

_____

_____

HOW I'M FEELING

☺ 😐 ☹

DATE _____   MO TU WE TH FR SA SU

- - - - - - - -   I SLEPT ____ HOURS LAST NIGHT   - - - - - - - -

TODAY I ATE _____

BREAKFAST
_____
_____
_____
_____

LUNCH
_____
_____
_____
_____

DINNER
_____
_____
_____
_____

TOTAL: CALORIES: [_____]

— SNACKS —

_____

WATER INTAKE ☐ ☐ ☐ ☐ ☐ ☐ ☐ __ TOTAL OZ.

EXERCISE/ACTIVITY
_____
_____
_____
_____

NOTES
_____
_____

HOW I'M FEELING
☺ ☺ ☹

DATE _____ MO TU WE TH FR SA SU

- - - - - - - -   I SLEPT ____ HOURS LAST NIGHT   - - - - - - - -

TODAY I ATE _____

BREAKFAST
_____
_____
_____

LUNCH
_____
_____
_____
_____

DINNER
_____
_____
_____
_____

TOTAL: CALORIES: [_____]

—— SNACKS ——

WATER INTAKE ⊔ ⊔ ⊔ ⊔ ⊔ ⊔ ⊔ __ TOTAL OZ.

EXERCISE/ACTIVITY
_____
_____
_____
_____

NOTES
_____

HOW I'M FEELING
☺ 😐 ☹

DATE _____   MO TU WE TH FR SA SU

| - - - - - - - -   I SLEPT ____ HOURS LAST NIGHT   - - - - - - - - |

TODAY I ATE _____

BREAKFAST
_____
_____
_____
_____

LUNCH
_____
_____
_____
_____

DINNER
_____
_____
_____
_____

TOTAL: CALORIES: [_____]

— **SNACKS** —

_____

| WATER INTAKE ⊔ ⊔ ⊔ ⊔ ⊔ ⊔ ⊔ __ TOTAL OZ. |

EXERCISE/ACTIVITY
_____
_____
_____
_____

NOTES   **HOW I'M FEELING**
_____
_____   ☺   ☺   ☹

DATE _____ MO TU WE TH FR SA SU

- - - - - - - - I SLEPT ____ HOURS LAST NIGHT - - - - - - - -

TODAY I ATE _____

BREAKFAST
_____
_____
_____
_____

LUNCH
_____
_____
_____
_____

DINNER
_____
_____
_____
_____

— SNACKS —

TOTAL: CALORIES: [_____]

WATER INTAKE ⊔ ⊔ ⊔ ⊔ ⊔ ⊔ ⊔ __ TOTAL OZ.

EXERCISE/ACTIVITY
_____
_____
_____
_____
_____

NOTES   HOW I'M FEELING
_____   ☺ 😐 ☹
_____

DATE _____ MO TU WE TH FR SA SU

┌───┐
│ - - - - - - - - I SLEPT ____ HOURS LAST NIGHT - - - - - - - - │
└───┘

TODAY I ATE _____

BREAKFAST

_____
_____
_____
_____

LUNCH

_____
_____
_____
_____

DINNER

_____
_____
_____
_____

┌─────────────────┐
│ —— SNACKS ——   │
│   │
│   │
│   │
│   │
│   │
│   │
│   _____ │
└─────────────────┘

TOTAL: CALORIES: [_____]

┌───┐
│ WATER INTAKE ⊔ ⊔ ⊔ ⊔ ⊔ ⊔ ⊔   __ TOTAL OZ. │
└───┘

EXERCISE/ACTIVITY

_____
_____
_____
_____

NOTES   **HOW I'M FEELING**

_____   ☺ ☺ ☹
_____

DATE _____   MO TU WE TH FR SA SU

- - - - - - - - | I SLEPT ____ HOURS LAST NIGHT | - - - - - - - -

TODAY I ATE _____

BREAKFAST
_____
_____
_____
_____

LUNCH
_____
_____
_____
_____

DINNER
_____
_____
_____
_____

TOTAL: CALORIES: [_____]

—— SNACKS ——

WATER INTAKE 🥛🥛🥛🥛🥛🥛🥛 __ TOTAL OZ.

EXERCISE/ACTIVITY
_____
_____
_____
_____
_____

NOTES   HOW I'M FEELING
_____   ☺ 😐 ☹

DATE _____   MO TU WE TH FR SA SU

- - - - - - - -   I SLEPT ____ HOURS LAST NIGHT   - - - - - - - -

TODAY I ATE _____

BREAKFAST
_____
_____
_____

SNACKS

LUNCH
_____
_____
_____

DINNER
_____
_____
_____

TOTAL: CALORIES: [_____]

WATER INTAKE 🥛🥛🥛🥛🥛🥛 __ TOTAL OZ.

EXERCISE/ACTIVITY
_____
_____
_____
_____

NOTES
_____
_____

HOW I'M FEELING

☺   😐   ☹

DATE _____ MO TU WE TH FR SA SU

- - - - - - - - I SLEPT ____ HOURS LAST NIGHT - - - - - - - -

TODAY I ATE _____

BREAKFAST
_____
_____
_____
_____

LUNCH
_____
_____
_____
_____

DINNER
_____
_____
_____
_____

TOTAL: CALORIES: [_____]

— SNACKS —

WATER INTAKE ⬚⬚⬚⬚⬚⬚⬚ ____ TOTAL OZ.

EXERCISE/ACTIVITY
_____
_____
_____
_____

NOTES
_____
_____

HOW I'M FEELING

☺ 😐 ☹

DATE _____   MO TU WE TH FR SA SU

- - - - - - - -   I SLEPT ____ HOURS LAST NIGHT   - - - - - - - -

TODAY I ATE _____

BREAKFAST
_____
_____
_____
_____

LUNCH
_____
_____
_____
_____

DINNER
_____
_____
_____
_____

—— SNACKS ——

_____

TOTAL: CALORIES: [_____]

WATER INTAKE 🥛🥛🥛🥛🥛🥛🥛 __ TOTAL OZ.

EXERCISE/ACTIVITY
_____
_____
_____
_____

NOTES
_____
_____

HOW I'M FEELING
☺ 😐 ☹

DATE _____   MO TU WE TH FR SA SU

- - - - - - - -   I SLEPT ____ HOURS LAST NIGHT   - - - - - - - -

TODAY I ATE _____

BREAKFAST
_____
_____
_____
_____

LUNCH
_____
_____
_____
_____

DINNER
_____
_____
_____
_____

TOTAL: CALORIES: [_____]

— SNACKS —

WATER INTAKE 🥛🥛🥛🥛🥛🥛🥛 __ **TOTAL OZ.**

EXERCISE/ACTIVITY
_____
_____
_____
_____
_____

NOTES
_____

HOW I'M FEELING

☺ 😐 ☹

DATE _____   MO TU WE TH FR SA SU

- - - - - - - -   **I SLEPT ____ HOURS LAST NIGHT**   - - - - - - - -

TODAY I ATE _____

BREAKFAST
_____
_____
_____
_____

LUNCH
_____
_____
_____
_____

DINNER
_____
_____
_____
_____

TOTAL: CALORIES: [_____]

—— **SNACKS** ——

WATER INTAKE ⬜⬜⬜⬜⬜⬜⬜ __ **TOTAL OZ.**

EXERCISE/ACTIVITY
_____
_____
_____
_____

NOTES
_____
_____

HOW I'M FEELING
☺ 😐 ☹

DATE _____ MO TU WE TH FR SA SU

- - - - - - - - I SLEPT ____ HOURS LAST NIGHT - - - - - - - -

TODAY I ATE _____

BREAKFAST
_____
_____
_____
_____

—— **SNACKS** ——

LUNCH
_____
_____
_____
_____

DINNER
_____
_____
_____
_____

TOTAL: CALORIES: [_____]

WATER INTAKE ⎕ ⎕ ⎕ ⎕ ⎕ ⎕ ⎕ __ **TOTAL OZ.**

EXERCISE/ACTIVITY
_____
_____
_____
_____
_____

NOTES
_____

HOW I'M FEELING
☺ 😐 ☹

DATE _____   MO TU WE TH FR SA SU

- - - - - - - -   I SLEPT ____ HOURS LAST NIGHT   - - - - - - - -

TODAY I ATE _____

BREAKFAST
_____
_____
_____
_____

LUNCH
_____
_____
_____
_____

DINNER
_____
_____
_____
_____

TOTAL: CALORIES: [_____]

—— SNACKS ——

WATER INTAKE ▯ ▯ ▯ ▯ ▯ ▯ ▯ __ TOTAL OZ.

EXERCISE/ACTIVITY
_____
_____
_____
_____

NOTES
_____
_____

HOW I'M FEELING
☺ 😐 ☹

DATE _____   MO   TU   WE   TH   FR   SA   SU

- - - - - - - -   **I SLEPT ____ HOURS LAST NIGHT**   - - - - - - - -

TODAY I ATE _____

BREAKFAST
_____
_____
_____
_____

LUNCH
_____
_____
_____
_____

DINNER
_____
_____
_____
_____

TOTAL: CALORIES: [_____]

— SNACKS —

WATER INTAKE ⬜⬜⬜⬜⬜⬜⬜ __ **TOTAL OZ.**

EXERCISE/ACTIVITY
_____
_____
_____
_____
_____

NOTES
_____

HOW I'M FEELING
☺   😐   ☹

DATE _____ MO TU WE TH FR SA SU

- - - - - - - -   I SLEPT ____ HOURS LAST NIGHT   - - - - - - - -

TODAY I ATE _____

BREAKFAST
_____
_____
_____
_____

LUNCH
_____
_____
_____
_____

DINNER
_____
_____
_____
_____

TOTAL: CALORIES: [_____]

— SNACKS —

_____

WATER INTAKE ⊔⊔⊔⊔⊔⊔⊔ __ TOTAL OZ.

EXERCISE/ACTIVITY
_____
_____
_____
_____

NOTES
_____
_____

HOW I'M FEELING
☺ ☻ ☹

DATE _____   MO TU WE TH FR SA SU

- - - - - - - -   I SLEPT ____ HOURS LAST NIGHT   - - - - - - - -

TODAY I ATE _____

BREAKFAST

_____

_____

_____

_____

LUNCH

_____

_____

_____

_____

DINNER

_____

_____

_____

_____

—— **SNACKS** ——

TOTAL: CALORIES: [_____]

WATER INTAKE 🥛🥛🥛🥛🥛🥛🥛 __ TOTAL OZ.

EXERCISE/ACTIVITY

_____

_____

_____

_____

_____

NOTES

_____

_____

HOW I'M FEELING

☺ 😐 ☹

DATE _____   MO TU WE TH FR SA SU

- - - - - - - -   I SLEPT ____ HOURS LAST NIGHT   - - - - - - - -

TODAY I ATE   _____

BREAKFAST
_____
_____
_____
_____

LUNCH
_____
_____
_____
_____

DINNER
_____
_____
_____
_____

TOTAL: CALORIES: [_____]

—— SNACKS ——

WATER INTAKE 🥤🥤🥤🥤🥤🥤 __ TOTAL OZ.

EXERCISE/ACTIVITY
_____
_____
_____
_____

NOTES
_____
_____

HOW I'M FEELING
☺ 😐 ☹

DATE _____   MO TU WE TH FR SA SU

- - - - - - - -   **I SLEPT ____ HOURS LAST NIGHT**   - - - - - - - -

TODAY I ATE _____

BREAKFAST
_____
_____
_____
_____

LUNCH
_____
_____
_____
_____

DINNER
_____
_____
_____
_____

TOTAL: CALORIES: [_____]

— **SNACKS** —

WATER INTAKE ⊔⊔⊔⊔⊔⊔⊔ __ **TOTAL OZ.**

EXERCISE/ACTIVITY
_____
_____
_____
_____
_____

NOTES   **HOW I'M FEELING**
_____   ☺ 😐 ☹
_____

DATE _____   MO TU WE TH FR SA SU

- - - - - - - -   I SLEPT ____ HOURS LAST NIGHT   - - - - - - - -

TODAY I ATE _____

BREAKFAST

_____

_____

_____

_____

LUNCH

_____

_____

_____

_____

DINNER

_____

_____

_____

_____

TOTAL: CALORIES: [_____]

— SNACKS —

WATER INTAKE ⬚⬚⬚⬚⬚⬚⬚ __ TOTAL OZ.

EXERCISE/ACTIVITY

_____

_____

_____

_____

NOTES

_____

_____

HOW I'M FEELING

☺ ☺ ☹

DATE _____   MO TU WE TH FR SA SU

| - - - - - - - -   I SLEPT ____ HOURS LAST NIGHT   - - - - - - - - |

TODAY I ATE _____

BREAKFAST
_____
_____
_____
_____

LUNCH
_____
_____
_____
_____

DINNER
_____
_____
_____
_____

TOTAL: CALORIES: [_____]

—— **SNACKS** ——

WATER INTAKE 🥛🥛🥛🥛🥛🥛🥛 __ **TOTAL OZ.**

EXERCISE/ACTIVITY
_____
_____
_____
_____
_____

NOTES   **HOW I'M FEELING**
_____
_____   ☺ 😐 ☹

DATE _____ MO TU WE TH FR SA SU

-------- I SLEPT ____ HOURS LAST NIGHT --------

TODAY I ATE _____

BREAKFAST
_____
_____
_____
_____

┌─────── SNACKS ───────┐

LUNCH
_____
_____
_____
_____

DINNER
_____
_____
_____
_____

_____

TOTAL: CALORIES: [_____]

WATER INTAKE ▯ ▯ ▯ ▯ ▯ ▯ ▯ __ TOTAL OZ.

EXERCISE/ACTIVITY
_____
_____
_____
_____
_____

NOTES   HOW I'M FEELING
_____   ☺ ☺ ☹
_____

DATE _____   MO TU WE TH FR SA SU

- - - - - - - -   **I SLEPT ____ HOURS LAST NIGHT**   - - - - - - - -

TODAY I ATE   _____

BREAKFAST
_____
_____
_____
_____

LUNCH
_____
_____
_____
_____

DINNER
_____
_____
_____
_____

TOTAL: CALORIES: [_____]

—— **SNACKS** ——

WATER INTAKE 🥛🥛🥛🥛🥛🥛🥛 __ **TOTAL OZ.**

EXERCISE/ACTIVITY
_____
_____
_____
_____
_____

NOTES   **HOW I'M FEELING**
_____   ☺ 😐 ☹
_____

DATE _____ MO TU WE TH FR SA SU

- - - - - - - -   I SLEPT ____ HOURS LAST NIGHT   - - - - - - - -

TODAY I ATE _____

BREAKFAST
_____
_____
_____
_____

LUNCH
_____
_____
_____
_____

DINNER
_____
_____
_____
_____

TOTAL: CALORIES: [_____]

—— SNACKS ——

_____

WATER INTAKE ⊔⊔⊔⊔⊔⊔⊔ __ TOTAL OZ.

EXERCISE/ACTIVITY
_____
_____
_____
_____

NOTES   HOW I'M FEELING
_____
_____   ☺ ☺ ☹

DATE _____   MO TU WE TH FR SA SU

- - - - - - - -   I SLEPT ____ HOURS LAST NIGHT   - - - - - - - -

TODAY I ATE _____

BREAKFAST
_____
_____
_____
_____

LUNCH
_____
_____
_____
_____

DINNER
_____
_____
_____
_____

TOTAL: CALORIES: [_____]

— SNACKS —

WATER INTAKE   [ ] [ ] [ ] [ ] [ ] [ ] [ ]   __ TOTAL OZ.

EXERCISE/ACTIVITY
_____
_____
_____
_____
_____

NOTES
_____

HOW I'M FEELING
☺ 😐 ☹

DATE _____ MO TU WE TH FR SA SU

- - - - - - - - I SLEPT ____ HOURS LAST NIGHT - - - - - - - -

TODAY I ATE _____

BREAKFAST

_____

_____

_____

_____

— SNACKS —

LUNCH

_____

_____

_____

_____

DINNER

_____

_____

_____

_____

TOTAL: CALORIES: [_____]

WATER INTAKE ⊔ ⊔ ⊔ ⊔ ⊔ ⊔ ⊔ __ **TOTAL OZ.**

EXERCISE/ACTIVITY

_____

_____

_____

_____

NOTES HOW I'M FEELING

_____   ☺ 😐 ☹

DATE _____   MO TU WE TH FR SA SU

- - - - - - - - **I SLEPT ____ HOURS LAST NIGHT** - - - - - - - -

TODAY I ATE _____

BREAKFAST
_____
_____
_____
_____

LUNCH
_____
_____
_____
_____

DINNER
_____
_____
_____
_____

TOTAL: CALORIES: [_____]

—— **SNACKS** ——

WATER INTAKE ⊔ ⊔ ⊔ ⊔ ⊔ ⊔ ⊔ __ **TOTAL OZ.**

EXERCISE/ACTIVITY
_____
_____
_____
_____
_____

NOTES
_____

HOW I'M FEELING
☺ 😐 ☹

DATE _____ MO TU WE TH FR SA SU

- - - - - - - - I SLEPT ____ HOURS LAST NIGHT - - - - - - - -

TODAY I ATE _____

BREAKFAST

_____
_____
_____
_____

—— SNACKS ——

LUNCH

_____
_____
_____
_____

DINNER

_____
_____
_____
_____

TOTAL: CALORIES: [_____]

WATER INTAKE ⊔ ⊔ ⊔ ⊔ ⊔ ⊔ ⊔ __ **TOTAL OZ.**

EXERCISE/ACTIVITY

_____
_____
_____
_____

NOTES

_____
_____

HOW I'M FEELING

☺ ☺ ☹

DATE _____   MO TU WE TH FR SA SU

- - - - - - - -   I SLEPT ____ HOURS LAST NIGHT   - - - - - - - -

TODAY I ATE _____

BREAKFAST
_____
_____
_____
_____

LUNCH
_____
_____
_____
_____

DINNER
_____
_____
_____
_____

TOTAL: CALORIES: [_____]

—— SNACKS ——

WATER INTAKE ☐ ☐ ☐ ☐ ☐ ☐ ☐ __ TOTAL OZ.

EXERCISE/ACTIVITY
_____
_____
_____
_____

NOTES   **HOW I'M FEELING**
_____
_____   ☺ 😐 ☹

DATE _____ MO TU WE TH FR SA SU

┌───┐
│ - - - - - - - -   **I SLEPT ____ HOURS LAST NIGHT**   - - - - - - - - │
└───┘

TODAY I ATE _____

BREAKFAST

_____
_____
_____
_____

LUNCH

_____
_____
_____
_____

DINNER

_____
_____
_____
_____

—— SNACKS ——

_____

TOTAL: CALORIES: [_____]

┌───┐
│ **WATER INTAKE** ⊔ ⊔ ⊔ ⊔ ⊔ ⊔ ⊔ __ **TOTAL OZ.** │
└───┘

EXERCISE/ACTIVITY

_____
_____
_____
_____

NOTES

_____
_____

HOW I'M FEELING

☺ 😐 ☹

DATE _____ MO TU WE TH FR SA SU

| - - - - - - - - I SLEPT ____ HOURS LAST NIGHT - - - - - - - - |

TODAY I ATE _____

BREAKFAST
_____
_____
_____
_____

LUNCH
_____
_____
_____
_____

DINNER
_____
_____
_____
_____

TOTAL: CALORIES: [_____]

—— SNACKS ——

WATER INTAKE 🥛🥛🥛🥛🥛🥛🥛 __ TOTAL OZ.

EXERCISE/ACTIVITY
_____
_____
_____
_____
_____

NOTES
_____
_____

HOW I'M FEELING
☺ 😐 ☹

DATE _____ MO TU WE TH FR SA SU

- - - - - - - - **I SLEPT ____ HOURS LAST NIGHT** - - - - - - - -

TODAY I ATE _____

BREAKFAST
_____
_____
_____
_____

LUNCH
_____
_____
_____
_____

DINNER
_____
_____
_____
_____

TOTAL: CALORIES: [_____]

—— **SNACKS** ——

WATER INTAKE 🥛🥛🥛🥛🥛🥛🥛 __ **TOTAL OZ.**

EXERCISE/ACTIVITY
_____
_____
_____
_____

NOTES
_____
_____

HOW I'M FEELING

☺ 😐 ☹

DATE _____   MO   TU   WE   TH   FR   SA   SU

| - - - - - - - - | I SLEPT ____ HOURS LAST NIGHT   - - - - - - - - |

TODAY I ATE _____

BREAKFAST
_____
_____
_____
_____

LUNCH
_____
_____
_____
_____

DINNER
_____
_____
_____
_____

TOTAL: CALORIES: [_____]

—— **SNACKS** ——

WATER INTAKE 🥛🥛🥛🥛🥛🥛🥛 ___ **TOTAL OZ.**

EXERCISE/ACTIVITY
_____
_____
_____
_____
_____

NOTES
_____
_____

HOW I'M FEELING

🙂 😐 🙁

DATE _____   MO TU WE TH FR SA SU

- - - - - - - -   I SLEPT ____ HOURS LAST NIGHT   - - - - - - - -

TODAY I ATE _____

BREAKFAST
_____
_____
_____
_____

┌─── **SNACKS** ───┐

LUNCH
_____
_____
_____
_____

DINNER
_____
_____
_____
_____

TOTAL: CALORIES: [_____]

WATER INTAKE ⊔⊔⊔⊔⊔⊔⊔ __ **TOTAL OZ.**

EXERCISE/ACTIVITY
_____
_____
_____
_____
_____

NOTES   **HOW I'M FEELING**
_____
_____   ☺ 😐 ☹

DATE _____   MO TU WE TH FR SA SU

- - - - - - - -   I SLEPT ____ HOURS LAST NIGHT   - - - - - - - -

TODAY I ATE _____

BREAKFAST
_____
_____
_____
_____

LUNCH
_____
_____
_____
_____

DINNER
_____
_____
_____
_____

TOTAL: CALORIES: [_____]

—— **SNACKS** ——

WATER INTAKE 🥛🥛🥛🥛🥛🥛🥛 __ **TOTAL OZ.**

EXERCISE/ACTIVITY
_____
_____
_____
_____
_____

NOTES
_____

HOW I'M FEELING
☺ 😐 ☹

DATE _____   MO TU WE TH FR SA SU

- - - - - - - -   I SLEPT ____ HOURS LAST NIGHT   - - - - - - - -

TODAY I ATE _____

BREAKFAST
_____
_____
_____
_____

LUNCH
_____
_____
_____
_____

DINNER
_____
_____
_____
_____

TOTAL: CALORIES: [_____]

— SNACKS —

WATER INTAKE 🥛🥛🥛🥛🥛🥛🥛 __ TOTAL OZ.

EXERCISE/ACTIVITY
_____
_____
_____
_____

NOTES
_____

HOW I'M FEELING

☺ 😐 ☹

DATE _____   MO   TU   WE   TH   FR   SA   SU

--------   **I SLEPT** ____ **HOURS LAST NIGHT**   --------

TODAY I ATE _____

BREAKFAST
_____
_____
_____
_____

LUNCH
_____
_____
_____
_____

DINNER
_____
_____
_____
_____

— SNACKS —

TOTAL: CALORIES: [_____]

WATER INTAKE ▢ ▢ ▢ ▢ ▢ ▢ ▢ ___ **TOTAL OZ.**

EXERCISE/ACTIVITY
_____
_____
_____
_____
_____

NOTES   **HOW I'M FEELING**
_____
_____   ☺   😐   ☹

Made in the USA
Middletown, DE
30 December 2021